Asthma: Your Quick G Treatment

ISBN-13: 978-1482533705
ISBN-10: 1482533707

GW00374607

Copyright Notice

ASTHMA: YOUR QUICK GUIDE TO UNDERSTANDING AND TREATMENT

Richard Threllin

Contents

What is Asthma?

Asthma is one of the world's most common diseases, but many people don't really know much about it.

This chronic lung disease is characterized by inflammation and narrowing of your airways, which bring about coughing, tightness in the chest, shortness of breath, and wheezing.

The coughing that accompanies asthma is usually experienced either in the early morning or at night.

Although asthma can affect you no matter how old you are, sufferers usually begin experiencing its symptoms during childhood.

It is estimated that there are about 300 million people who suffer from asthma all over the world and about 30% of sufferers are children.

The importance of getting asthma diagnosed and treated properly lies in the fact that the disease causes thousands of deaths all over the world each year.

Add to that the fact that the number of asthma cases has risen significantly in recent years and you'll understand why it is indeed important to learn as much as you can about this disease.

A better understanding of asthma can be gained with some knowledge about how your airways normally work.

Airways are basically the tubes where air passes out of and into your lungs.

These tubes are inflamed in people with asthma and the inflammation causes the airways to swell and become very sensitive.

When you inhale certain substances, the sensitive airways can react immediately, causing the surrounding muscles to tighten. As a result, the airways are narrowed and less air flows into your lungs.

This will then bring on the usual asthma symptoms and is the reason why most asthma sufferers are said to be allergic to dust and strong odours.

Inflamed airways also react strongly to climate changes and cause asthma symptoms to occur.

Although there are some common symptoms of the disease, you need to bear in mind that each person may experience a different set of symptoms.

In the same way, the intensity of asthma attacks may also vary from one sufferer to the next.

There are times when asthma symptoms are relatively mild and just disappear on their own.

But, there are also instances when the symptoms just become more intense, in which case you are said to be experiencing a flare-up.

It is important to get asthma symptoms treated as soon as you experience them so as to avoid worsening, especially since flare-ups often require emergency care and may even lead to death.

The reasons for asthma attacks haven't exactly been confirmed yet, but doctors are pointing at both environmental and genetic factors as contributors to the condition.

The fact that no direct cause has been identified also means there isn't any cure yet for asthma.

The best thing you can do, with the guidance of your doctor, is treat your symptoms and manage the disease such that it doesn't hamper your daily routines.

The good news is that with the right combination of medication, behaviour adjustments, and environmental changes, you can still enjoy a productive life even when you have asthma.

What's important is for you to build a strong relationship with your doctor and work actively to manage your condition.

Types of Asthma

If you suffer from asthma or know someone who does, then you understand how scary the symptoms of this disease can be.

The good thing is that medical advancements have helped identify the different types of this disease and understanding what type of asthma you're suffering from could be the first step towards getting it treated in the most effective way.

Exercise-induced Asthma

This type of asthma, as the name implies, can be triggered by physical exertion such as exercise.

Although most of those who have asthma experience their symptoms to some degree when they physically exert themselves, there are those whose symptoms are triggered only by exercise.

With this type of asthma, you're likely to experience shortness of breath five to twenty minutes after you start exercising.

You could also start coughing and wheezing.

You'll have to ask your doctor if using an inhaler before you exercise can help you keep the symptoms under control.

Cough-variant Asthma

This type of asthma is characterized by coughing as its predominant symptom. Asthma is, in fact, one of the most common causes of cough these days, but it almost always goes undiagnosed or undertreated.

Physical exertion and respiratory infections are among the usual triggers of this type of asthma.

If you start experiencing a persistent case of coughing, it is best to consult your doctor right away.

You may have to undergo a series of asthma tests and it may even be advisable for you to consult a lung specialist to make sure you get properly diagnosed.

Occupational Asthma

This type of asthma is brought about by triggers in the workplace.

If you suffer from this type of the disease, then you can expect your symptoms to act up only on the days when you're at work.

Many of those who have this type of asthma experience nasal congestion, runny nose, or eye irritation.

Coughing is also more common than wheezing in this case.

The most common types of work that can bring on this type of asthma are farming, animal breeding, painting, woodworking, hairdressing, and the nursing profession.

Nocturnal Asthma

This type of asthma is also known as night time asthma and is one of the most common types of this disease.

Your chances of experiencing asthma symptoms normally increase at night when you sleep, since the disease is largely influenced by the normal circadian rhythms.

The problem is that wheezing, coughing, and shortness of breath are also most dangerous at night.

In fact, studies have shown that most asthma-related deaths actually happen at night.

It is believed that this is because of your reclined position and the fact that your airways are cooled and you're more exposed to allergens when you sleep.

Be sure to work closely with your doctor in treating this type of asthma and remember that it's not just important to take the right medication in this case, but also to make sure you take your meds at the right times.

Knowing what type of asthma you're suffering from gets you one step closer to finding the most effective treatment option.

So, the moment you start experiencing asthma symptoms of any kind, be sure to consult your doctor right away and get yourself properly diagnosed.

Triggers and Risk Factors

If you've recently been diagnosed with asthma, you'd certainly do well to learn what the common triggers and risk factors for the disease are.

This knowledge will help you avoid doing things or getting near objects that may cause an asthma attack.

To begin with, you may want to take note of conditions that are known to cause asthma.

These conditions include a history of the disease in your family. If someone in your family has been diagnosed with the disease, then it's best to get yourself checked as well, whether you've started experiencing symptoms or not.

It is also a good idea to get yourself checked if you had some sort of lung infection as a child.

Those who've had respiratory infections as a child and those who live in areas where there are plenty of allergens should also get checked for asthma.

If you frequently contract animal dander, then you should also be prepared to develop asthma.

If you're a smoker or are frequently exposed to second-hand smoke, then you're also in danger of getting asthma.

Other than these conditions, there are also factors that usually trigger asthma attacks and you'd also do well to bear these in mind and do your best to avoid them.

Remember that asthma is a chronic disease, which means that once you develop it, you will always have it in you.

But, you will only experience asthma attacks when your asthma triggers are present. The exact cause of the disease itself, however, is yet to be determined.

In the same way, medical practitioners are still trying to come up with a cure for the condition.

At this time, the best that you can do is to avoid your asthma triggers as much as you can.

Take note that the triggers are likely to differ from one asthma sufferer to the next.

Air pollution is among the most common asthma triggers.

When polluted air enters your airways, it usually causes irritation, inflammation, and swelling.

The swelling will then lessen the amount of air that enters your lungs and consequently lead to the wheezing that characterizes an asthma attack.

If you've been diagnosed with asthma, you'd do well to avoid living in areas with factories that pollute the air.

The hair of your pets is also likely to trigger an asthma attack, so it may be wise not to have pets at home.

If letting your pet go is too painful, then you should make sure your pets are always clean and that they spend more time out of the house.

You should also avoid letting your pet sleep on your bed or in your bedroom.

Dust mites, molds, and cockroach droppings are also possible asthma triggers.

This makes it important for you to keep your home clean by regularly vacuuming and mopping all surfaces.

You should also change your pillow covers and mattresses frequently so as to protect yourself from dust mites.

And because molds typically grow in humid conditions, you would do well to use a humidifier or air conditioner at all times.

Drastic weather changes have also been known to trigger asthma attacks.

Since weather isn't something you can control, it's best to always have your medication on hand for these instances.

What's most important is for you to determine what your specific triggers are and then do your best to avoid them.

Symptoms

Asthma is a chronic disease that's characterized by inflammation in your bronchial tubes and an increase in the sticky secretions in those tubes.

Asthma sufferers typically begin experiencing symptoms when their airways become swollen or tighten due to the increase in mucus production.

Tightness and pain in the chest, shortness of breath, coughing, and wheezing are the most common symptoms of the disease.

But, each asthma sufferer will have a different set of symptoms from another.

The severity of the symptoms and the time of day when you usually experience them can also vary from one person to the next. Furthermore, the severity can vary from one asthma attack to another.

There are times when you may not experience any symptoms for long periods and then you'll suddenly suffer from a severe attack.

For some people, though, asthma symptoms have become part of their daily struggles.

Still, other sufferers only experience symptoms when they physically exert themselves or when they have viral infections or at certain times of day.

In most cases, asthma attacks are relatively mild and the sufferer's airways open up after a few minutes.

Though they're less common, severe attacks typically last longer and often require medical attention.

Even if your asthma is mild, though, it's advisable to treat it immediately so as to avoid a worsening of symptoms.

It is equally important for you to learn of the early signs that typically occur right before an asthma attack.

These warning signs usually begin before the actual asthma symptoms occur and they're the first signs that your condition is getting worse.

These warning signs are seldom so severe as to interrupt your normal daily activities.

But, it's important to recognize these signs so you can either stop an asthma attack in its tracks or at least prevent the attack from worsening.

These early signs include frequent coughing, particularly at night, a feeling of extreme tiredness during exercise, wheezing after physical exertion, irritability, sore throat, nasal congestion, sneezing, headaches, and trouble getting to sleep.

Once you start experiencing these warning signs, you may take your medication to prevent the onset or at least minimize the severity of an asthma attack.

In an actual asthma attack, triggers cause the muscles surrounding your airways to tighten.

At the same time, the triggers cause your airways to swell and the lining to produce more mucus than it normally does.

These factors then combine to bring on the usual asthma symptoms such as wheezing, coughing, and shortness of breath.

Other than these symptoms, you may also experience rapid breathing, retractions in your chest and neck muscles, chest pain, anxiety or panic attacks, blue lips and fingernails, pale and sweaty face, or talking difficulties.

Whatever symptoms you exhibit, be sure to treat them as soon as you realize that you're having an attack or about to have one.

The severity of your symptoms could increase very rapidly if you don't seek immediate treatment.

An attack could even become life-threatening, which is why immediate treatment is a must.

Unusual Symptoms

Wheezing is perhaps the most common sign that you're suffering from asthma. Aside from this, however, the disease may also have some unusual symptoms.

One of these other symptoms is a dry and persistent hacking cough.

Additionally, you may also experience breathing difficulties and tightness in the chest when you develop asthma.

Some asthma sufferers are also known to sigh constantly, breath rapidly, and have difficulty focusing on things. Unusual asthma symptoms also include anxiety and fatigue.

To make things even more complicated, not only are there a lot of things that may indicate asthma, but the symptoms you experience may also vary from one asthma attack to the next.

For example, you may start out experiencing symptoms only at night.

On succeeding asthma attacks, however, you may experience symptoms during the day and these symptoms may be triggered by a variety of factors.

Asthma triggers include smoke, dust, cold air, infections, acid reflux, and even some medications.

Bear in mind that there are also health conditions accompanied by symptoms similar to those of asthma, which is why you need to have yourself properly diagnosed.

One of the most common asthma triggers is exercise.

Those who suffer from exercise-induced asthma often experience shortness of breath, tightness in the chest, and coughing.

Symptoms typically occur about ten minutes after exercise begins or ten minutes after you complete an activity that requires physical exertion.

In some cases, however, the onset of symptoms doesn't start until about four to eight hours after you've completed your exercise session.

This type of asthma is most common in kids and young adults. The good thing is that it is both preventable and treatable.

Another factor that's commonly associated with asthma is chronic cough.

Though this can indeed be one of the most common asthma symptoms, bear in mind that there are other possible causes of chronic cough.

Aside from asthma, chronic cough may also be brought about by pneumonia, bronchitis, postnasal drip, acid reflux, lung cancer, heart disease, smoking, and some medications used for hypertension treatment.

If your cough lasts for longer than three weeks, you may want to be checked for these conditions to be sure that you're properly diagnosed.

If your chronic cough is caused by asthma, you may first it experience it after you've had a cold or suffered an infection in your upper respiratory tract.

Chronic cough as an asthma symptom may also begin as a tickling in your throat.

Some people who have asthma can have a coughing fit even after doing something as simple as laughing.

Coughing may occur at night or at any time of the day and sometimes even without an obvious trigger.

If your coughing is brought on by asthma, then cough drops, cough suppressants, and antibiotics aren't likely to do you any good. What you need is proper asthma treatment.

If you suffer from any of the symptoms mentioned above, be sure to get a clear diagnosis by seeing your doctor immediately.

This is especially important if you're experiencing a combination of the above-mentioned symptoms. Your health isn't something you can just take for granted.

Diagnosis

The necessary first step towards the proper treatment and management of asthma is getting properly diagnosed.

After your doctor has determined that you indeed have asthma and identified what type of asthma you're suffering from, he can start discussing treatment and management options with you.

Following your doctor's advice on this matter will help you continue living a productive and active lifestyle.

One of the biggest problems associated with diagnosing asthma is the fact that the disease often doesn't exhibit any obvious symptoms while you're in your doctor's office.

For example, you may have been coughing non-stop and wheezing for a couple of weeks, but when you get to your doctor's clinic, you've stopped wheezing and coughing completely.

When you get back home and at a time when asthma is farthest from your mind, you could suddenly start coughing and wheezing again.

There are several things that may trigger asthma symptoms.

These things include weather changes, seasonal pollen, viral infections, allergies, sudden stress, and even exercise.

Other than these potential triggers, there are also things that can worsen your symptoms and increase the severity of your asthma.

These things include smoking, environmental allergies, and sinusitis.

Once you've developed asthma, remember that you don't necessarily experience the symptoms on a daily basis.

In fact, some sufferers can go for months without suffering from a single asthma attack or even from the mildest of symptoms.

This makes it even more difficult to diagnose the disease. This also makes it very important for you to do your homework before you even visit your doctor.

Take note of all your symptoms and triggers as well as the severity of the attacks and the time of day you experience the symptoms.

Keeping a record can help your doctor arrive at an accurate diagnosis.

Needless to say, an accurate diagnosis is crucial to appropriate and effective treatment.

Your doctor plays a very important role in the proper diagnosis and treatment of your condition.

Because of this, you'll have to work closely with him and establish a strong relationship built on trust.

You should be able to treat your doctor like a friend on whom you rely for support, particularly when your symptoms start to cause some real worry.

If it makes you feel any better, you could ask your family doctor to refer you to an asthma specialist with ample experience in treating the disease.

A qualified specialist will begin by obtaining your medical history and asking you for some detailed information as regards your symptoms and triggers.

He is also likely to ask how you feel, what your normal activity level is, what your diet normally consists of, what your work environment and home situation is like, and if you have any family history of asthma.

During this evaluation phase, you shouldn't hesitate to discuss all of your symptoms and ask any questions you may have.

It would help a lot if you get everything clear even before your doctor begins your physical examination and laboratory testing.

An open discussion with your doctor will also make it a lot easier for you to work together on an effective treatment and management plan.

Getting Tested for Asthma

When you start exhibiting symptoms that may be caused by asthma, it is best to consult your doctor immediately for testing and diagnosis.

There are a number of key tests that are used for diagnosing asthma.

Some of these tests measure your lung function whereas others determine if you have allergies to pollen and other particles as well as to specific foods.

Blood tests will also be conducted in order for your doctor to get a picture of your health in general.

There are also more specific tests for measuring your immunoglobulin levels, since people with allergies typically have higher levels of this antibody.

These tests are meant not only to determine the presence of asthma, but also of possible coexisting conditions.

Your doctor can only prescribe medications once proper diagnosis is made.

Chest X-Ray

This is perhaps the most basic physical exam you'll have to undergo.

Although it doesn't specifically determine whether you have asthma, a chest X-ray is used to rule out anything else that may be causing your symptoms, such as broken bones or bronchitis.

This test will also allow your doctor to view the condition of your lungs, which will give him an initial idea as to whether your symptoms may indeed be caused by asthma.

Lung Function Test

If your doctor sees a possibility for asthma in the chest X-ray results, he will proceed to make an assessment of your lung function.

Methacholine challenge and spirometry are the most commonly conducted lung function tests for diagnosing asthma.

Spirometry is usually conducted first. This is a basic breathing test that gauges the speed with which you can blow air from your lungs.

It is meant to determine if there is any obstruction in your airways.

If the results of this test are inconclusive, then your doctor may recommend a methacholine challenge test.

Allergy Tests

Allergies have been known to trigger or worsen asthma symptoms.

It is for this reason that your doctor may conduct allergy testing as well.

If results show that you have allergies, then treatment may focus on addressing not only the asthma symptoms, but also your allergies.

Evaluation of Your Sinuses

If you have sinusitis, your asthma may become more difficult to manage. Bacteria normally grow when your sinuses are blocked and fluid fills it. As a result, your sinuses get infected and become inflamed.

If your doctor suspects that your sinuses are infected, he may conduct a CT scan.

If results show that you do have sinusitis, antibiotics will likely be prescribed in order to relieve not just the sinusitis itself, but also your asthma symptoms.

Based on the physical exam and test results, your doctor will know if your condition is indeed asthma. If it is, the next step would be to determine its severity in order to arrive at a viable treatment plan.

Asthma can be mild and intermittent, mild yet persistent, moderate and persistent, or severe and persistent.

Remember to work closely with your doctor in drawing up a treatment and management plan.

Participating actively in your own treatment is essential to its effectiveness.

Questions You Should Ask Your Doctor

If you suspect that you may have asthma, then you definitely need to consult the right kind of doctor to make sure he understands the nature of the condition and the treatment options that are available to you.

You may want to consider consulting an allergist, since most allergists specialize not only in allergies, but also in asthma and allergic asthma.

An internist would also be a good choice, since internists specialize in diseases that have to do with your internal organs.

These doctors typically undergo three years of training after they graduate from medical school.

Another option would be for you to consult either a pulmonologist or a pulmonary rehabilitation therapist.

A pulmonologist is trained specifically for treating respiratory diseases and some of them even undergo training to get board certification for critical-care medicine.

A pulmonary rehabilitation therapist, on the other hand, is a duly-trained nurse or respiratory therapist.

Not only can he offer support for managing asthma, but he is also equipped to provide you with all the necessary information on how to alleviate your symptoms, handle a therapeutic exercise program, avoid stress, and improve your lung function.

Of course, it's not enough for you to find the right kind of doctor who can help you manage your condition.

You also need to ask the right questions to make sure you have a clear and complete understanding of your condition and the treatment you'll be going through.

The first questions you need to ask once you're diagnosed with asthma, of course, has to do with what this disease is and what its causes are.

The answers to these questions will give you a general idea of what you're dealing with and will help equip you for managing it properly.

You'd also do well to discuss your current lifestyle and daily routines with your doctor and then ask him if there are any changes you need to make so as to reduce the likelihood of asthma attacks.

Other than that, it would also be advantageous for you to learn about the tests you'll have to go through in order to monitor your condition.

You should also ask for a demonstration on how to use an asthma inhaler to make home treatment a lot easier.

You may also want to ask about some home remedies and alternative treatment options that may be used along with your medications.

Many people think exercise is bad for asthma sufferers and that may be true to some extent.

But, some form of exercise may actually be helpful, as it can strengthen your lungs and improve its function.

It is therefore a good idea for you to ask your doctor about a good exercise program that can complement your treatment program.

Finally, you'd do well to ask your doctor about any support group he may know of.

It can be a bit difficult to handle any medical condition on your own and even if you have your family's support, it's an entirely different thing to have the support of other people who know exactly what you're going through simply because they're going through the same thing.

Preventing Asthma Attacks

Once you're diagnosed with asthma, that you're going to have to deal with the condition for the rest of your life.

There is no known cure for it and the best that you can do is get relief from its symptoms and prevent asthma attacks from occurring and disrupting your daily routines.

So, what exactly can you do to prevent asthma attacks or at least lessen their severity?

Here are some tips:

1. If you have carpets at home, get the m removed. Carpeting is one of the favourite areas of dust, dust mites, and other allergens. These allergens can easily get back to the surface and circulate in the air, thus triggering an asthma attack.

    By removing all carpets from your home, you make the surfaces easier to clean and rid yourself of a considerable amount of asthma triggers.

y pets like cats and dogs,
say goodbye to them as
d dander are among the
irritants that trigger
, so no matter how much
ets, you'll have to let them
want to make your
condition worse.

3. Take advantage of probiotics. These are bacteria normally found in your gut. Studies have shown that these bacteria are very useful for reducing allergic symptoms and inflammation. For this reason, asthma sufferers are often advised to take probiotics in the form of cultured yogurt. You may want to do the same.

4. Reduce your intake of meat, shellfish, and egg yolk. These foods are known to contain arachidonic acid, which has been shown to cause inflammation. Reducing your intake of these foods is expected to reduce the incidence of inflammation in your lungs as well. And in case you do suffer from inflammation, the severity will likely be reduced if you avoided these foods.

5. Avoid going to place where cigarette smoke abound. It goes without saying that cigarette smoke is hazardous to your condition. The good thing is that cigarette smoking has been banned in public places in many states. This definitely reduces your worries in case you have to go to restaurants and bars for whatever reason. However, if such a ban isn't being implemented in your area just yet, you'll have to be very careful when going out to make sure you don't suffer the consequences of inhaling too much cigarette smoke.

6. Learn some relaxation techniques. Studies have shown that stress can bring on an asthma attack and increase the severity of one. Other studies have also shown that taking advantage of relaxation techniques on a regular basis, and most especially when you feel symptoms about to act up, effectively holds an asthma attack at bay.

These are the basic things you can do to prevent asthma attacks and help make your treatment and management program more effective.

Of course, it would be best for you to discuss every detail of your asthma treatment with your doctor.

As long as you take an active role in the management of your condition, it shouldn't cause too much disruption in your life.

Natural Remedies

Are you looking for natural remedies that can help relieve your asthma symptoms?

If so, then you're not alone.

A lot of asthma sufferers tend to look for natural remedies. These remedies typically include dietary supplements, herbs, massage therapy, acupuncture, homeopathy, botanicals, biofeedback, and chiropractic therapy.

Home remedies may also include adjustments in your diet to ensure proper nutrition.

Remember, though, that there's just a limited number of studies so far as regards alternative asthma treatment, so you may want to do a lot of research before taking advantage of any natural treatment method.

As mentioned above, a number of plants, herbs, and dietary supplements have been suggested as natural treatments for asthma. These include Vitamin E, Vitamin C, and Omega-3 fatty acids.

Your doctor isn't likely to recommend them because of a lack of definitive studies, but many people who've used them swear by their effectiveness.

Those who recommend acupuncture claim that this form of alternative therapy helps improve your breathing.

Still, others swear by biofeedback, which involves learning how to control your heart rate.

Where diet and nutrition is concerned, the main thing is to avoid foods that may trigger allergy attacks.

And because stress is said to worsen asthma, you may also want to try relaxation techniques like yoga.

When you mention herbs to anyone, they're likely to think "natural" and automatically assume that it's safe to use for whatever condition they may have.

Bear in mind, though, that a lot of herbs actually haven't gone through the necessary amount of testing for safety.

Moreover, herbal supplements and medication aren't regulated as strictly as other forms of medicine.

In the case of herbal medication for asthma, take note that some herbs used for this purpose have been shown to interact with other medications.

This makes it even more important for you to discuss every single medication you plan to take, natural or otherwise, with your doctor.
Since most of the natural asthma remedies currently being sold aren't properly regulated, it can be a bit difficult to know exactly which ones are safe without asking your doctor.

Some of these supplements may even interact negatively with the medication your doctor has prescribed, thus worsening your condition.

In case you've started taking a natural asthma remedy and you end up with negative side effects like nausea, vomiting, anxiety, rapid heartbeat, diarrhea, skin rashes, or insomnia, you need to stop taking the supplement immediately and then tell your doctor about it.

When choosing natural remedies for asthma, it pays to choose your brands very carefully.

The brands most people trust and which have been around for many years usually offer the safest and most effective remedies.

You'd also do well to go with brands that clearly list the scientific and common name of the main ingredient as well as any other ingredient that may have been included in the formulation.

The batch and lot number, dosage guidelines, potential side effects, expiration date, and manufacturer's name and address should also be listed.

Transparent brands are often the most trustworthy. Don't just trust commercial claims. Do your own homework to ensure the safety of any natural asthma remedy you choose to take.

Air Cleaners

According to asthma-related studies, most homes around the world have the kind of air that's filled with pollutants of all kinds. These pollutants include dust, bacteria, mold spores, and chemical vapors.

And these pollutants have been shown to be related to an increase in the incidence of asthma symptoms acting up in recent years.

Does this mean you need to buy an air purifier for every room in your house?

If you can afford to do so, then that would indeed be a good idea.

The problem is that this solution is far too expensive for most people.

It's a good thing, then, that there's another solution known as an air cleaning system for your entire house.

To get the best results, you'd do well to get an air cleaning system that's attached directly to your furnace ducts or air conditioner. It's also advisable to choose a system that includes a considerable amount of activated carbon as well as HEPA filters.

These filters are capable of removing about 99.97% of pollutants and the activated carbon takes care of any chemical vapors, odors, and gases in the air, thus leaving the air within your house considerably cleaner than before.

Needless to say, this can make a huge difference in your life. It'll help you sleep better at night and reduce your risk of suffering from asthma attacks.

The best air cleaning systems typically cost anywhere between $1200 and $1500.

This may seem very expensive, but when you consider that a portable air purifier costs between $600 and $700 each, you'll realize that it's a lot more affordable than buying one purifier for each of the rooms in your house.

Another advantage of having one system for the entire house is that it saves you from having to drag an air cleaner from one room to another just to make sure the air is free from allergens that may trigger your asthma symptoms.

Remember that not all home air cleaning systems are the same. You'll have to take a number of things into consideration to make sure you get the best system for your needs.

The first step is for you to make sure you get a system from a well-reputed manufacturer.

Check testimonials regarding the brand and the specific product you're considering.

Check ratings from independent reviews as well. The more people trust a brand, the more reason you have to choose it over other brands.

Another thing you need to ensure is that the system has a HEPA filter, rather than a HEPA-style filter. HEPA-style filters don't work as well as HEPA filters do.

You should also make sure the air cleaning system you choose isn't equipped with electronic sensors that automatically turn the system on or off.

You'll naturally want your air cleaner working whenever your air conditioning is turned on.

You never know how much vapour, gas, or other pollutants are permeating the air in your home so it's a good idea to keep cleaning the air around you.

Soon after you start using a home air filter system, you'll be sure to notice a marked improvement in your breathing as well as increased comfort when you sleep.

More importantly, your asthma symptoms will start acting up much less frequently.

Nutrition and Asthma

If you want to keep breathing easily and stay active despite having asthma, then you'll definitely need to take an active role in managing your condition.

Among other things, you'll have to learn what diet and exercise have to do with keeping your symptoms at bay.

You should also learn how to keep your stress and anxiety levels down, as these are also among the common triggers for asthma attacks.

Although there isn't a specific diet recommended for asthma sufferers and there are no foods that are known to reduce the inflammation of the airways that's characteristic of asthma, it is often advised for you to ensure proper nutrition.

After all, everyone can benefit from a good diet, right?

This becomes even more important when you take into consideration the fact that obesity has been linked to severe cases of asthma.

This should drive home the importance of maintaining a healthy weight at all times.

Even doctors hold the suspicion that some foods may directly impact your condition.

Of course, further research is needed in order to gain a better understanding of the direct link between diet and asthma.

Right now the rule of thumb is that you should avoid all foods that trigger allergies, since allergic reactions typically trigger asthma attacks.

A lot of researchers believe that changing diets play a major role in the increase of asthma cases that has been observed in recent years.

As people eat more processed food and less fresh fruits and vegetables, we may be inadvertently increasing our risk for developing asthma.

There are already several studies that suggest this association and more studies are currently being conducted to get more definitive answers.

To be more specific, studies suggest that those who take in higher doses of Vitamin C, Vitamin E, beta-carotene, Omega-3 fatty acids, flavonoids, selenium, and magnesium are less likely to suffer from asthma.

It isn't really clear, however, whether a deficiency of these nutrients can actually cause people to develop asthma.

To add to the confusion, some medical professionals have tried using certain vitamins and minerals to treat some asthma patients, but the treatment has proven unsuccessful.

This has led some researchers to believe that the health benefits one gains actually comes not from a particular vitamin or mineral, but from the interaction among these vitamins, minerals, and antioxidants that occur naturally in fresh foods.

Whatever the direct link between diet and asthma is, one thing remains certain: If your diet doesn't include the necessary nutrients, then you become more susceptible to all kinds of illnesses, including asthma.

This makes it highly advisable for you to eat plenty of fresh fruits and vegetables.

You'd also do well to take in foods that are rich in Omega-3 fatty acids. These foods include tuna, salmon, sardines, and flaxseed.

You should also avoid taking in trnas-fats and foods rich in Omega-6 fatty acids, since there's evidence that these substances can worsen serious health conditions like heart disease and asthma.

You've probably heard some people say you are what you eat. If you eat healthy, therefore, you *are* healthy.

Asthma and Exercise

One of the most common questions people have when they get diagnosed with asthma is whether it's still safe to engage in regular exercise.

Well, when you consider the fact that asthma treatment is primarily focused on helping you lead a productive and healthy lifestyle, then you'll understand that exercise is, in fact, an essential part of an effective treatment program.

 If your asthma symptoms are disrupting your daily routines, then it would be best for you to talk to your doctor about adjustments in your treatment program that may be necessary to get relief from asthma even while exercising.

It is generally believed that activities involving short periods of exertion work best for people with asthma.

These activities include gymnastics, wrestling, volleyball, and baseball. Sports like basketball, soccer, field hockey, and distance running may not be recommended, since these activities normally involve long periods of exertion, which asthma sufferers are unable to tolerate that well.

It's also advisable for you to avoid sports played in cold conditions like ice hockey, ice skating, and cross-country skiing.

You may, however, engage in skating or skiing for short periods of time.

A better alternative would be for you to take up swimming, which is an excellent activity not only for asthma treatment, but also for maintaining overall fitness. Biking, walking, running on a treadmill, and aerobics are also recommended activities for asthma sufferers.

There are things you need to consider and steps you need to take in order to ensure that your asthma is still under control even as you engage in exercise.

First of all, you should never forget to use any pre-exercise inhaler your doctor may recommend before you start any physical activity that may be considered a form of exercise.

Second, you should warm up properly before performing your actual exercises and then be sure to cool down right after.

If you're exercising during cold weather, be sure to exercise indoors or wear a mask over your mouth and nose, should you choose to exercise outdoors.

If you suffer from allergic asthma, be sure to avoid exercising outdoors where there's plenty of pollution or a high pollen count. It is also best to limit your exercise when you're suffering from viral infections such as a cold.

Finally, you should remember to exercise only at a level that's appropriate for your physical capabilities.

Remember that it's important to maintain an active lifestyle for your mental and physical health.

Asthma shouldn't be a reason for you to avoid engaging in regular exercise.

As long as you get properly diagnosed and are able to map out an effective treatment and management program with your doctor, you should be able to continue enjoying the benefits of a workout routine even as you live with asthma.

If you do experience asthma symptoms during exercise and you don't get relief from your inhaler, stop exercising immediately and call your doctor for assistance.

Bear in mind that your treatment program will only work if you coordinate closely with your doctor at all times.

Living with Asthma

Even if you've been living with asthma symptoms for some time and you feel that you can handle it well enough on your own, you should still seek some professional help. You could choose to visit your doctor or better yet, an asthma specialist.

You may even choose to seek help from other people who suffer from the condition as well.

It is understandable for you to feel a little anxious and maybe even overwhelmed by the constant bouts of wheezing and shortness of breath that's common with asthma.

Having asthma can indeed be very stressful and the irony is that you need to avoid stress, as it can worsen the condition.

This makes it even more important for you to learn some techniques that can make it a lot easier to live with the condition.

Stress may not be among the causes of asthma, but there is a definite link between the two. As mentioned earlier, asthma can make life more stressful and stress can make the condition a lot more difficult to manage.

Even the stress you're normally subjected to at work can worsen your asthma symptoms. It is therefore important for you to learn how to manage stress better so as to reduce the incidence and severity of your asthma symptoms.

It may also be necessary to set up a daily schedule such that you're able to accomplish everything that needs to be done without feeling overwhelmed.

Take note that the longer you let your breathing problems go untreated, the likelier you are to notice that it gets worse when you're stressed.

You may also start experiencing other problems such as sleeping difficulties, nocturnal asthma, and constant fatigue. This constant fatigue can lead to the inability to engage in exercise as well as poor physical fitness.

Pretty soon, you'll also notice that you're suffering from concentration difficulties, which can ultimately lead to poor work performance.

And because you're no longer sleeping very well, you'll likely become irritable and you may even begin to withdraw from the activities you normally enjoy simply because you feel too tired to engage in them.

Some people even suffer from depression as a result of uncontrolled asthma symptoms.

The good news is that you can live with asthma without succumbing to its symptoms. The first step towards accomplishing this is learning how to adjust your stress response.

You'll need to actively set goals that'll help you manage the stress that you deal with on a regular basis. This allows you to make sure that you deal with stress in a healthy manner and in such a way that doesn't worsen your breathing problems.

You may notice that when you start getting stressed, your anxiety level increases and your asthma symptoms act up.

If you ignore this, it becomes a vicious cycle that soon leads to a complete downward spiral. This is why it's important for you to learn more about the connection between stress, anxiety, and asthma.

Talk to your doctor or therapist about it and about ways of properly dealing with stress and reducing anxiety in an effort to better manage your asthma symptoms.

Getting Support

Asthma is considered among the world's most common diseases and it affects about one in ten children and one in 20 adults all over the world.

The good thing about this is that it means the condition is relatively well-understood by medical professionals.

Although there is yet no known cure for the condition and medical professionals haven't yet identified the exact cause of the inflammation of airways that brings on asthma, the fact that it is well-understood means a number of methods are in place that allows you to continue living a productive lifestyle even when you've been diagnosed with the condition.

If you have indeed been diagnosed with asthma, then it's important for you to get support. Of course, the people around you (most especially your family) can provide the primary circle of support.

These people include your co-workers and friends and you should make sure they're properly informed about what to do in case of an asthma emergency.

More importantly, they should be aware that there are ways to keep asthma properly managed and under control.

For this reason, it is important for you to give a copy of your asthma treatment and management plan to your family, friends, and colleagues.

When you prepare copies of your treatment and management plan to give to your support group, you have to make sure it includes the contact information of your doctor or asthma therapist.

Additionally, it should indicate all of the medications you're taking along with dosage instructions and how often you need to take each medicine.

You should also list down everything that triggers your asthma symptoms, be they substances or behaviours.

This way, your family and friends can help make sure you don't get into situations that may increase your risk of suffering from an asthma attack.

The asthma action plan you give out to your support group also has to contain a description of your asthma control zones.

The green zone is your best control zone, the yellow zone refers to instances when symptoms are worsening, and the red zone refers to your medical alert zone.

Your control zones are determined by readings on a peak flow meter, which is a device used to measure breathing.

When the peak flow readings are between 80% and 100%, you're still within your green zone; when the readings are between 50% and 79%, you're within your yellow zone; when the peak flow readings go lower than 50%, you already require immediate medical attention.

There is perhaps no need to explain why your support group needs to learn about your control zones.

Of course, your family, friends, and colleagues aren't your only sources of support when you're dealing with asthma.

And indeed they shouldn't be because support groups are very valuable for people living with a chronic condition like asthma.

Among other things, they provide you with an environment wherein you can learn other alternatives where living with asthma is concerned.

People who have been living with the condition for years can share the approaches they take with you.

At the same time, you can share the approaches you're taking with others who may benefit from it.

More importantly, support groups provide you with strength from knowing that you're not facing asthma alone.

Printed in Great Britain
by Amazon

49843277R00059